The Path *To* Health

*A manual for proper
care of the human body.*

DR. RICHARD L. ROBLES, DC

Foreword by Dr. Christi L. Wiley, MD

ISBN: 1490435026
ISBN-13: 9781490435022
Library of Congress Control Number: 2013911448
CreateSpace Independent Publishing Platform
North Charleston, South Carolina

"The winding road of life will take you on many unexpected journeys, we must remember to take heed of the boundaries along the road in order to stay on course to our desired destinations along the way."

by Dr. Richard L. Robles, DC

INTENDED USE

The contents of this book and/or e-book are intended for informational purposes only. Any medical information in this book is intended as general information only and should not be used to diagnose, treat, cure, or prevent any disease. The goal of this book is to present general information about care of the body and offer suggestions that can be used to improve general health.

DISCLAIMER

Statements contained in this book and/or e-book have not been evaluated by the Food and Drug Administration. The information and recommendations outlined in this book are not intended as a substitute for personalized medical advice; the reader of this book should see a qualified healthcare provider. This information is not intended to diagnose, treat, cure, or prevent any disease. This information is not to be used as a substitute for appropriate medical care and consultation, nor should any information in it be interpreted as prescriptive in nature. Any person who suspects a medical problem or disease should consult their physicians for proper treatment and guidance. The information here is provided for educational and/or general informational purposes only, which is implicitly not to be construed as medical advice. No claims guarantees, warranties, or assurances are implied or promised. This book and e-book are for information only and their contents are the opinion of the author and should not replace the advice of the reader's physician.

CONTENTS

ACKNOWLEDGEMENTS

I dedicate this book to my loving wife and children. Without their love, support, and life lessons I would not have found my higher purpose. Thank you to my parents for their love and encouragement. My brothers, sisters, and extended family who have all supported me in their own special ways. Thank you to all of my mentors and colleagues, most of whom will never know the impact they have had on my journey, with special thanks to Dr. Tim Francis, Dr. Victor Frank, Dr. Datis Kharrazian, Dr. Michele Cohen, Dr. Aaron Wilkerson, Dr. Michael Johnson, Dr. Andy Barlow, and especially Dr. Christi Wiley. Many thanks to Jan Bezanson for her editing prowess, Paul Robles for his technical abilities, and Ray Robles for his unwaivering support. Thank you to all of my patients who choose to work with me and let me practice on them, and from who I have learned so many clinical lessons from and for.

FOREWORD

It's no secret that chiropractic and allopathic doctors are not exactly on the same page when it comes to strategies on the treatment of various ailments. In fact, it would be safe to say that most of the time they are polar opposites.

With all the differing opinions on the process, it's easy to overlook that both practitioners have a common goal – the health and well being of the patient. This commonality is what initially sparked my interest in Dr. Robles' book, The Path to Health. I discovered that his book is essentially a universal primer for the care of the human body, and before I even finished reading it, I found myself applying its principles in my own practice.

For years, I have been an advocate for my patients, encouraging them to be proactive and partner in their health. Finally, there is a book that provides a step by step guide to get your health back. A book that challenges you to accept responsibility and take action, rather than passively sit back and watch as the chronic diseases of our society run a muck.

The Path to Health explains the basic physiology of the human body in a way that is easy to understand and apply. It bucks the tide of conventional thoughts about food and nutrition and answers some of the basic questions about what we should put in our body and how we should treat our body. We make sure our cars get the correct gasoline. You wouldn't dream of putting 87 octane in a car that calls for premium, but somehow we don't question or care about what we put in our bodies, or even where it came from. Dr. Robles helps us to understand why these things are important.

As practitioners, we all tell our patients the path to good health is to eat right and exercise. In response, we see an annoyed or bewildered look as they wonder "how?" We all know that the mantra is easier said than done, but sometimes time or fund of knowledge and resources are lacking, and the patient and the physician end the visit dissatisfied. This book is a quick resource to not only answer the question of how, but why. So, read on, and start living the healthy lifestyle you were meant to have.

Dr. Christi L. Wiley, MD

INTRODUCTION

"Well, Mr. and Mrs. Wilkerson, you're just going to have to learn to live with some of those symptoms, take your medications, and try to work on improving your health. Your labs look good, there will not be any further treatment at this time. We'll keep an eye on things, and see how you do," said Doctor X.

This scenario is far too common these days. *You'll just have to learn to live with some of those symptoms! Take your medicine, and we'll keep an eye on things!* They grew up in a house that kept them warm, had three square meals each day, finished school, and started a family. They are getting older and, of course, since they are getting older they should expect that things just don't work the same as they used to, or that it will take a little longer to get going. They should expect that some diseases just come with age.

STOP! That is not the way it should be.

This manual is designed to set the record straight on diet, nutrition, and health on the most basic level. Why is it that humans have been around for thousands of years, in some of the harshest living conditions, yet we have "experts" on diet and health telling us that we need some new wonder drug, or special protein powder, or the extract from a plant on top of a Himalayan mountain in order to stave off disease or in order to be healthy? Have we lost touch with the information that our ancestors discovered through trial and living? Do we now think that we know better than they did in all regards, despite the inherent wisdom passed on to us? There must be a common ground between the inherent wisdom of our ancestors and present day health knowledge, or a *basic, structured Path toward human health.* This Path, when we follow it, should improve our health, and when we don't follow that Path we will suffer (to some varying extent) the consequences. To put it simply, *when we do not live a life that promotes health, our body will let us know by sending out a signal that it needs help in the form of a symptom.* The speed at which these consequences or symptoms occur depends on how far off the Path of Health we have strayed. The quickest and most severe symptoms are usually designed to keep us alive and stop us from engaging in activities that might kill us immediately. The chronic, long-lasting symptoms typically result from straying off the Path to Health for an extended period of time.

We have slowly been robbed of our health and most of us are not even aware of it. Our health has been hijacked, and we have been left vulnerable. We have been left to suffer for long periods of time with chronic diseases, often living longer, but not healthier. The basic knowledge of what our body needs to be strong and vibrant has been lost. It has been replaced with commercial information, that is bought by whoever can pay the most money for advertisements, or "research" that supports their latest "health" product. Information that has not stood the test of time and cannot support the heavy task of building a healthy body. Under the stress of the modern diet and lifestyle, our health eventually deteriorates and we develop symptoms. What do we do? How do we get back something that we did not know we had lost?

We have to be re-educated on the very basics of how our body works. Consider that *we are taught from a very young age that our body requires energy, and that our food is the primary source of our energy supply.* This concept represents some of the oldest, and most basic, fundamental knowledge we will ever need to know about our body. Yet, there is more to the food story than that, even though that is all of the story that most of us like to hear or want to know. *We need more than just energy from our food, we need to incorporate that energy into our body and use it for nourishment.* The idea that we are just eating to get energy is a basic, foundation concept that is important, but needs to be augmented as our ability to understand more complex ideas increases. Here is an example of what I mean: *Remember back to the time you were learning to read.* First, you learned the letters of the alphabet, but that was not the end of the lesson, you did not stop there.

You then learned to combine the letters to form words and sentences. Next you to put the words and sentences into order to make paragraphs... and finally the sky was the limit. Now, imagine if you had never learned to put the letters together to build words, sentences, paragraphs, essays, poems, dissertations, books, etc.

Unfortunately, our education system often teaches us *just* the "alphabet," when it comes to diet, nutrition, and health. Our basic knowledge of these systems should be increased by our education system and then expanded by our doctors. These two resources of health knowledge are failing to get solid basic information out to the general population. This sad fact can be exemplified by the rate of increase in the incidences of chronic diseases in our country, despite advances in medications, surgeries, physical therapy, nutritional supplement popularity, etc. The information available to our educational institutions and doctors has become an instrument used to make money. The pharmaceutical industry and biotechnology companies provide a great example of corporations that are in the business of health research. These companies are in the business of producing research that leads directly to new products, and consequently new profits. Therefore, it is by no stretch of the imagination that their interests would lie in proving only the worth of their products and protecting their bottom line. Research that is truly directed toward the advancement of our health would investigate both the positive and negative aspects with equal scrutiny. However, their profits are not determined by the health of their consumers, but by the market share of their products. These are the companies who make the most money on our health (really large amounts of money) and have a vested interest in an undereducated, disempowered society. The buyers and sellers of health information want you to be confused about the most basic health concepts. This confusion allows people, who may only be experts in name, to tell you what you need. You must need this *new* product or medication, or that *new* health food or supplement in order to *be healthy*. There is always a reason why they are advertising their expertise to you and why it is done at the expense of you feeling empowered to help yourself. That ends here. That is why this book has been written.

Follow the advice in this manual and you will be able to manage your health. If you have lost your health, in one way or another, you can use this manual to help aid your recovery and slow future loss of health. This journey is not always easy, because you must rethink many concepts that have undermined your basic understanding of your body. Along this journey, you will realize that you "kinda knew" that you should treat your body according to this manual, and at the end you will also have a basic understanding of *why* you should do it.

THE BASICS

"We are charged to take care of our bodies so that we have optimum expression of our genetics passed on to us by our parents and onto our children after us."

We receive genes from our mother and father. We are the genetic expression of our parents. This unique combination of genetic material from our parents is what causes our expression of dark hair or light hair and dark eyes or light eyes. It determines the strength of our immune system and what allergies we will start life with, as well as our sensitivity to the world around us. In essence, our genes determine what our body's threshold is for the chemical, physical and emotional stress load, or toxic load, that we may experience in our life. They determine our breaking point to withstand these stressors and bear the burden of our toxic load. The capacity to withstand these stressors is different for each of us. The ability to adapt to stress is as unique as our fingerprints. This is why members of the same family, who grew up eating the same food, and had similar physical and emotional stress, can have significantly different lives when it comes to disease. This is because their ability to handle their toxic load, or the toxic load experienced by their mother (especially while she was pregnant), was different. So, one child may grow up with mild problems, and another in the same family may grow up with more severe problems. *How?*

Much of this has to do with the epigenetic influence on the genes we are born with. In addition to the genes we talked about earlier, we are born with genes that are not expressed outwardly, as well as genes that help us adapt to the environment we live in. Think of these genes like a light bulb. The light bulb only shines light once it has been turned on, or once the light switch has been flipped on. These genes may not be expressed at birth, but, can be activated or "switched on" as a response to the environment we live in. This is how humans have adapted to be able to live in such a wide variety of environments. The key point here is that these unexpressed genes are "switched on" in response to the world around us. The epigenetic influence can be thought of as a "light switch" that activates these genes and represents the interplay between the environment around us and the expression of our genetics.

So, how does this affect me? The "epigenetic light switch" functions differently in different people. For some, it may be a switch that is easily flipped, and for others, a big, metal lever that takes great effort over a long period of time to switch on. The difference in our body's ability to deal with the environmental stressors around us will determine whether or not the interactions of our epigenetics will activate a gene or cause an expression of a gene. When we have consistent stress on the body, the epigenetic influence on the genes that promote specific diseases within the body can be activated. This can contribute to, or account for, the expression of age-associated diseases, inflammatory arthritis, type I or II diabetes, thyroid disease, and many other common conditions.

We are charged to take care of our bodies so that we have optimum expression of our genetics passed to us by our parents and onto our children after us. Our society has evolved in ways that have removed our responsibility to take care of our bodies and allowed our focus to be shifted away from our health. Consider what health meant to people 3000 years ago. It was the determining factor in who was able to live longer, have more children, and who might die sooner. **Our advances in science, technology, and disease have given most of us the ability to live longer lives despite more abuse to our bodies.** Now is your chance to refocus your attention onto your life's purpose and get your health back!

WHAT TO EAT AND DRINK

"We want to get our food from sources that are as close to natural as possible, and the same rule applies to the preparation of our food."

There is a lot of information out there about what we should eat and why we should be eating it. Unfortunately, a lot of that information is wrong. It typically falls into one of four categories: information from flawed theories; information from flawed practice; both flawed theory and practice; or good information. When it comes to which foods to eat, the guideline is very simple. If you eat food that has not been changed from the way that it looked when it was walking around, or living in the ground, it will do more good than harm (except in rare occasions which will be discussed later). Let me be clear. Meat, fish, vegetables, and fruit will do more good than harm, and should be at the core of your diet.

Basic Rules of Eating:

1. *Eat breakfast or a morning snack within 30 minutes of waking up in the morning.*

2. *Each of your three main meals should contain vegetables and a protein source, with snacking*

occurring throughout the day (at least one snack in between each meal).

3. *Vegetables should be eaten in quantities that are equal to twice your intake of fruit. This does not mean to eat less fruit, in general, it means to eat more vegetables.*

There are two major areas where we need to increase our awareness:

1. Our food sources and preparation of food.

2. The way food affects our energy levels.

Redefining the four basic food groups will allow us to really get a sense of what to eat and where our food should come from. Let's start with the basic concept of *eating food that has not been changed from the way that it looked when it was walking around, or living in the ground.* This concept will help us combine food into the first two food groups. These food groups are listed as *Groups 1 & 2* in **Figure 1**. The first place to start making changes, or adjustments to what you allow yourself to eat, should be the elimination of packaged or boxed foods. These foods have changed shape from when they were harvested at least once. In many cases these foods have been changed so much, that you can hardly recognize it as something that once grew in the ground or walked around. The processing of a food has a direct effect on the nutritional value inherent to that same unprocessed food. This would include breakfast cereals, doughnuts, pasta, pastries, cookies, candy, TV-dinners, microwave burritos, chicken nuggets, etc. In general, these foods will fall into the foods listed in *Group 3 & 4* in **Figure 1**. That does not mean that you should only avoid them if they come in a box or package, but also if they are freshly prepared, because they will still contain many components that have been altered from their natural state. Care in the preparation of our food is one area where we stray from the course; our food sources are another.

Figure 1- *The four basic food groups*

Group 1	Group 2	Group 3	Group 4
Wild food sources, from a unpolluted environment	Organic Meat, Eggs, Vegetables, & Fruit	Conventional Meat, Vegetables, & Fruit	Processed Food
			Organic Tea
		Organic Grains	Organic Coffee
Organic Sustainably-Raised Vegetables, & Fruit	Fermented Conventional Foods	Organic Processed Food	Organic Sweeteners
Fermented Organic Foods	Organic nuts, beans, lentils, legumes	Farm-raised fish	Grains
Organic pasture-raised Meats & Eggs			
Wild-caught fish			

**Note: Organic coffee, tea, and sweeteners have been included in Group 4 due to the stimulatory effect of these items.

Our food sources have changed over the course of time to increase crop size and yields. This often has come at the expense of the nutrient quality of our food, along with the addition of numerous chemicals that have no place in our food or in our bodies. Many of the foods included in *Groups 3 & 4* of **Figure 1** have been altered at the source of production. Additionally, some crops have even had radiation exposure that not only changes the crop to optimize profits, but also changes them in ways that raise questions about whether or not we should even eat those crops (wheat is a good example). A trip to your local grocery store will illustrate this. All the produce is large and looks the same with little evidence that it was actually once in the ground, on a tree, or on a bush. This neat display at the grocery store comes at a price. That price is paid primarily by the stress incurred by our bodies to deal with processing the chemical laden produce; factory farmed meat, poultry, and fish; or the altered genetic structure of modern grains. We get beautifully packaged food that looks just like it does in the encyclopedia (or on Wikipedia), but those foods can often make a meal more stressful than healthy for our body. This is due to the change in the nutrient content and the increased activation of our immune system by these foods.

We want to get our food from sources that are as close to natural as possible, and the same rule applies to the preparation of our food. Ideally we want to eat our food with as little processing or changing of its form as possible. Therefore, raw food that is minimally processed is a goal to strive for. Raw food allows our bodies the opportunity to receive nourishment from unaltered proteins, carbohydrates, and fats, as well as the ability to use some of the natural enzymes and other nutrients contained in the food for the digestive process. This means that ingestion, digestion, absorption-assimilation, and elimination can occur at a rate and with a rhythm that will improve your health. That is if you have not significantly lost your health in some way, shape, or form. Loss of health will be covered later in this book, in the **Getting Your Health Back** section.

There are a few variables that complicate the intake of a raw food diet for many people. Consider that the average person today has high perceived or emotional stress, which causes a decrease in the availability of digestive acids and enzymes. These digestive acids and enzymes not only allow us to breakdown the foods into usable components, but they also serve a role in protecting our bodies from bacteria, viruses, and other contaminants that may be along for the ride. The high stress of modern society has a direct impact on our body's ability to digest properly. Therefore, the average American is not digesting food well. This allows for frequent exposures of our immune system to bacteria, viruses, parasites, as well as undigested proteins from food, which can begin to activate immune reactions in our body. As these immune reactions continue over a long period of time, they begin to negatively affect our health. As a result, we must cook our foods as an alternative form of protection, or avoid certain foods altogether.

Have you ever wondered why a bear or lion can eat raw meat, or drink from a stream without becoming ill, but the same cannot be said for humans? This is in part because the average person's body cannot adequately protect itself nor can it quickly restore balance to our systems. We are left to ingest cooked food, because our body may not be capable of digesting the contaminants in our food if it were raw. In other words, the average American is so far removed from the source of their meal and the food has been so heavily processed that the food is often tainted in ways that make eating the food in it's raw form unrealistic.

Fermented (not pickled) foods are a lost treasure, missing from most Americans' diets. Raw, fermented foods, such as sauerkraut, kefir, kimchi, kombucha, raw yogurt (unpasteurized), raw cheese, etc. play a vital role in maintaining the health of our digestive system. The processing required to ferment our food should not be confused with the processing involved in making your standard pasteurized products, pickled produce, or other packaged foods. The health benefits obtained from the conventional sources of foods such as yogurt, cheese and pickles are mostly eliminated by the process in which they are made. In general, you should limit your intake of pasteurized foods. Instead, search out and pay the extra cost, if necessary, for quality, clean, organic fermented foods.

A combination of the information contained in the **Basic Rules of Eating** and **Figures 1, 2, 3** will allow you to answer the question of: *What should I eat?*

As you progress through this manual, you will be reminded to go back to a basic, healthy diet. These three Figures will serve as the basic information to aid in building a foundation for your recovery from a wide range of symptoms, and to augment any care that you are currently under.

Figure 2 is designed to help establish an understanding of how much of our diet should come from each of the four food groups. The table is broken down into percentages, but can easily be translated into quantity of foods eaten over the course of a day.

***See the note underneath Figure 2.**

Figure 3 is designed to give you examples of foods that fall into different food categories. Such as meat, vegetables, and fruit. This list is not comprehensive of all possible fruits, vegetables, and meat sources, but should serve as a guide to help establish better eating habits. The foods listed in these categories are congruent with the foods listed in **Figure 6,** which will be discussed later.

Figure 2- *How much to eat of each food group*

	People with a heavy diagnosis	People diagnosed with a disease	People with Daily symptoms	No Daily Symptoms
Group 1	85%	80%	75%	70%
Group 2	15%	15%	23%	20%
Group 3	0%	5%	5%	5%
Group 4	0%	0%	2%	5%

**Note- *Another way to look at this chart is as follows: 70% means that 7 out of every 10 items you eat will come from Group 1, 20% means that 2 out of every 10 items you eat will come from Group 2, 5% means that 1 out of every 20 items you eat will come from Group 3, 5% means that 1 out of every 20 items you eat* will come from Group 4 for individuals with no daily symptoms. Therefore, most of the food you eat should come from groups 1 and 2 and very little should come from groups 3 and 4.

Figure 3- *Different types of Foods by category*

Animal Meat	Fish, eggs, beef, turkey, shellfish, chicken, game meats
Vegetables	Asparagus, artichoke, broccoli, cabbage, carrots, celery, collard greens, dandelion greens, garlic, kale, kohlrabi, leeks, lettuce, mustard greens, onions, parsley, potatoes, radish, rhubarb, rutabaga, salads, shallots, spinach, squash, sweet potatoes, turnips, water chestnuts, watercress, yams, zucchini
Fruit	Fresh apples, apricots, avocados, berries, cherries, grapefruit, grapes, lemons, oranges, peaches, pears, plums, nectarines, prunes, mango, melons, pineapple
Fermented Foods	Sauerkraut, kombucha, fermented coconut products, kimchi, fermented vegetables & fruit
Herbs and Spices	Anise, basil, bay leaf, black pepper, cilantro, coriander, cumin, garlic, ginger, lemongrass, mint, onion, oregano, parsley, rosemary, sage, sea salt, thyme, tumeric
Nuts & Seeds	Almonds, sunflower seeds, sesame seeds, walnuts, cashews, macadamia nuts, brazil nuts, pistachios
Beans & Legumes	Black beans, pinto beans, lentils, peas, kidney beans, azuki beans, butter beans
Grains	Rice, buckwheat, millet, sorghum, quinoa

Water

There is no life without water! These are words to live by. They have rung true throughout history, and at present, guide our future exploration of the universe. The body's water requirements are different for each person, however, there are two basic formulas which will help you narrow down your **ideal water intake:**

The first basic formula: **Drink 1 quart of water for every 50 lbs of body weight.**

The second basic formula: **Body weight divided in half equals the number of ounces you should drink.**

Your optimal water intake is usually in between the calculations from these two formulas (Remember 1 quart equals 32 ounces, and 1 gallon equals 4 quarts or 128 ounces).

Many people will have different water requirements, so these basic guides are a starting point to determine your needs. You will notice that you get a different amount of water for each formula. Most people will find that their intake should be somewhere in between the amounts determined by the two formulas. If you get thirsty during the day, your water intake is not adequate. If your urine is yellow as it comes out of your body (and the color change is not from taking supplements or medication), you may need to drink more water. The ideal water intake schedule is as follows: Adults: Drink 6 – 8 ounces of water upon rising, then drink 1-2 pints of water about 45-60 minutes before your major meal. Children: Drink 2 – 6 ounces of water upon rising, then drink 8 – 16 ounces of water about 45-60 minutes before your major meal. The majority of your water consumption should be *before* or *after* your meals, *not with* your meals. Keep in mind that you should drink water with your meals, however, just enough to satisfy your thirst during the meal.

What about other beverages? Ideally we should only consume water, however, other beverages often find their way into our cups. With that in mind, green tea can be consumed (ideally) at no more than one cup per day. Milk derived from nuts, rice, and coconuts are good sources of nutrition, if they do not contain additives, or sweeteners. Exclude all sodas, bottled juices, milk, coffee, and alcohol. (Please refer to **Figures 1, 2 & 6** for clarification)

Should I drink my water hot, warm, or cold? The temperature of your water does not matter in most cases. This also depends upon the weather. For example: If you are outside in cold weather, ice cold water may be an added stressor, rather than a source of refreshment. The same may be true of hot water in hot weather. Don't go out of your way to avoid cold water, as that is how it is found most abundantly in nature.

How much to eat.

We eat food to satisfy our body's requirements for energy and nourishment, however, there is one basic need that everyone should be aware of: **one of our only jobs each day is to eat enough of the** *right food to satisfy our energy needs throughout the day and store away enough energy to keep us alive throughout the night.* When we do that job daily, our body will thrive. When we don't do our job, more frequently than we do our job, our body will let us know with symptoms.

When we eat food, it is broken down into small pieces by our teeth, then into smaller pieces by the enzymes and acids in our bodies. One of these small pieces is glucose, a basic unit or molecule of sugar. This glucose will be moved into our blood stream (now considered blood sugar) and carried, along with oxygen and other nutrients, out for distribution into every part of our body to provide the fuel that makes our body work. One of the major signals that allows our body to bring this glucose into our cells to make energy is insulin. So, it is not only important for us to bring the glucose into our body by taking in enough food, but we have to listen to the signal from insulin to move the glucose into our cells to actually make the energy. This is the basic information that will allow us to figure out whether we are doing our job, which is: bringing in energy.

The two most important categories of symptoms to assess whether or not you are eating enough food and adequately bringing it into your cells for energy production are: symptoms of hypoglycemia and symptoms of hyperglycemia. Hypoglycemia is too little sugar in your blood, which will not allow your body to produce the energy necessary to fuel your body. You will usually find some or all of the symptoms in *Figure 4* are present when you tend towards hypoglycemia. Hyperglycemia is too much sugar in your blood, which will cause your body to use alternative means to remove the sugar from your blood, some of which actually cost your body energy. You will usually find some, or all, of the symptoms in *Figure 5* are present when you tend towards hyperglycemia. Please note that it is possible to have symptoms of both of these conditions which is called dysglycemia. Dysglycemia is the inability of the body to maintain steady levels of glucose in the blood or the inability to move it readily into the cells for energy production.

Figure 4- *Hypoglycemia or low blood sugar symptoms*

Irritability relieved by eating	Forgetfulness
Lightheaded/Dizziness relieved by eating	Headaches (especially behind the right eye)
Fatigue (mental and/or physical) relieved by eating	Salt cravings

Figure 5- *Hyperglycemia or high blood sugar symptoms*

Fatigue after a meal	Getting sleepy after a meal
Not being able to concentrate after a meal	Frequent urination
Frequent hunger	Frequent/Increased thirst

If you eat food that significantly increases the glucose/sugar in your blood, it becomes stressful on your body. Prolonged increase, or consistent fluctuations (such as eating a large breakfast and not eating again until dinner with a large dinner portion) will also cause your body to slowly lose the ability to adequately move the blood sugar into your cells to produce energy. When this happens, your body will have to spend energy to repackage and store the blood sugar, and this will often cause sleepiness and/or fatigue after a meal or other symptoms from *Figure 5*.

If you do not eat enough food to get a consistent supply of energy into your body, the first place to suffer is your brain. Your brain is the most oxygen and glucose dependent part of your body. This is because your brain cannot store oxygen or glucose in proper amounts to meet its needs. Therefore, it needs a constant supply of fuel (oxygen and glucose). When your brain does not get the required fuel you will experience hypoglycemic symptoms such as those mentioned above in *Figure 4*. These symptoms are primarily due to the inability of your brain to keep up with the demands you are putting on it without increased energy supplies on a consistent basis.

The type of food you eat has a direct influence on your body's ability to create energy. Think of your blood sugar like a fire burning inside of your body that is used to make energy. How you manage your fire will determine whether or not the flame is too high, too low, polluting your body with smoke, or burning just right. Eating fruit or vegetables would be like adding paper to your fire, it will burn quickly and brightly. Eating meat, fish, or other proteins is like placing wood on your fire, it will burn steadily over a longer period of time. It is stressful on your body if your fire burns too high, too low, or produces too much smoke. What types of foods create smoke and/or cause the fire to rise too high or too low? Processed food, pasta, most commercially available breads, pastries, candy, etc. can be likened to throwing plastic water bottles, or lighter fluid onto a fire. They will cause the fire to create smoke, give off strange gases, or burn excessively high and burn out quickly. These foods can be identified in *Groups 3 & 4* from ***Figure 1***. Those foods tend to cause more harm, or stress on your body, rather than improving your health. Especially from the energy production standpoint.

So, we must manage our energy production to stay healthy. In other words, manage your internal fire and you will stay warm and healthy. Think about what you are placing in your fire: paper, plastic, lighter fluid, or wood?

Remember, calories are only one small factor in choosing what to eat, and often not the most important factor. It is the advent of processed food and other goods that have created a need for the labeling of food. Over time, this has lead us to inappropriately value the calorie as the most important hallmark in our food choices and label reading.

Is what I'm eating hurting my body?

It is important to eat food for nourishment and it is equally important to avoid foods that actually hurt us, or hinder our body from functioning properly. Identification of food sensitivities is an integral part of figuring this out. Several of the staple foods in the Standard American Diet are some of the most common foods that we are sensitive to. Foods such as wheat, milk (dairy) products, soy, and corn can cause irritation to your body in ways that you may not even be aware. It is not uncommon for people to find that they have sensitivities to foods that they have eaten their entire life! Then, once they remove these foods from their diets, they find that many symptoms they did not relate to their diet vanish.

Here is why: Food sensitivities to items that are eaten everyday are often the spark that lights the fire of pain and disease. Imagine that multiple times a day you may be eating food that is causing your body to become sick, but you have been told by "health experts" that these same foods are "healthy" for you. This is what you need to know: Food sensitivities cause activation of your immune system, typically a delayed immune response, which can cause symptoms outside of your digestive tract. The hardest concept for people to understand about food sensitivities is that the most common symptoms are **not digestive!** This leaves most people with no idea that their symptoms are related to what they are eating.

Why hasn't your doctor talked to you about this? It's likely that your doctor does not know about the connection between food sensitivities and disease, "doesn't believe in it", or has not had the time to help you understand their impact on your health. Our health care system is designed to apply treatments to large volumes of people in short amounts of time. This limits your doctor's ability to stay current on research and educate the patient about their role in maintaining their health. The time to connect the dots between the combined effects of multiple stressors on our health and their impact on the development of disease simply does not have a place in our current health care system. This is especially true when the stressors are the very same remedies that health experts are touting as "healthy" solutions for chronic problems, or, when the very foods that we have been told are healthy, are actually making us sick.

So, how do you know if you have a food sensitivity?

The best method (it also tends to be the safest method) is through a blood test and an elimination diet. However, either one by itself will also give you valuable information. Either of these choices are best administered by a health professional who has experience in providing these tests and explaining the results. If you are in doubt about a food, it is best to leave it out. The consequences of being incorrect are not worth the stress on your body (which is also the reason why having a blood test first is important). **Your body's ability to determine whether or not something is "bad" for it is superior to our best lab tests.** Therefore, combining the blood tests with an elimination diet will tend to yield more information about your food sensitivities.

The value of the lab testing is that you will lessen the likelihood of inadvertently reintroducing foods that may worsen your condition. Additionally, it can be a great confirmation that you are doing the "right thing," and it will arm you with information that will help you answer questions about the changes you are making in your life to those around you.

It is important to discuss the similarities and differences between a food intolerance and a food sensitivity. They are both stressful to your body, but in a different ways. A food intolerance typically refers to a non-immune system mediated response to a food, often to a sugar or fat. Where a food sensitivity is an immune system response to one or more proteins in a particular food. Most people, and their doctors, tend to minimize the importance of both food sensitivities and a food intolerance. They are often written off as "normal" digestive problems, or something you may "outgrow." However, they can often be at the root of more serious health problems, that can only be resolved once the diet is adjusted to eliminate the problematic foods.

Once you have identified the foods you are sensitive to and removed them from your diet, it is time to review the other foods you should avoid. In general, the foods listed in **Figure 6** are foods to avoid to maintain or improve your health. Many of these foods hinder various body functions and can cause harm in your body. Additionally, artificial foods such as, hydrogenated oils, partially hydrogenated oils, food colorings, food by-products, natural flavors, artificial flavors, artificial sweeteners, natural sweeteners, GMO foods should all be avoided.

Figure 6- *What not to eat*

Any food that you are allergic to.	Any food that you are sensitive to.
Wheat & Gluten	Non-organic Corn
Pasteurized and/or conventional dairy	Non-organic Soy
Genetically Modified Foods- Non-organic corn, soy, sugar beets, alfalfa, canola, etc.	Peanuts
	Unfermented Cauliflower
Fastfood	Soda, carbonated drinks, alcohol
Hydrogenated oils, partially hydrogentated oils, trans fats	

***Note: Genetically Modified Foods (or GMO foods) have become widely used in conventional farming. The high percentage of convetionally farmed or non-organic corn, soy, sugar beets, alfalfa, & canola* *that are GMO make it reasonable to add those foods to the list of those that should be avoided.*

Some foods can cause low levels of inflammation in our bodies. This can be due to the type of food, how the food is prepared, or how often certain foods are eaten. Low levels of inflammation from inappropriate food choices for your body can build up over time to cause dysfunction in your body. Some of these foods that hinder the function of our body can often be foods that are thought of as healthy. This would include some of the foods in the nightshade family (tomatoes, potatoes, peppers, etc.), beans, lentils, and legumes. These foods can be difficult for some to digest and/or clear from our bodies. These foods should be rotated out of our diets to ensure they are not contributing to our internal inflammation levels.

Other foods that hinder your body function, and can cause harm in your body, are (most) conventionally farmed/produced products such as meat, fish, fruit, and vegetables. This is primarily due to the herbicides, pesticides, GMO feed, overcrowding, antibiotics, vaccines, pasteurization, etc. common place to conventional farming and production. Herbicide and pesticide residues are often absorbed by the plants we eat. When these plants are consumed by people, they can disrupt the function of hormones and enzymes in our bodies. Antibiotic residues can be found on plants and can also accumulate in the meat of the animals we eat. This can lead to increases in weight, dysbiosis, and also the development of antibiotic resistant bacteria. You will need to increase your awareness of these dietary stressors to more clearly define the boundaries of your path to health. Additionally, this information should help you understand the importance of choosing organic whenever possible.

MAINTAINING YOUR HEALTH

"Health is the optimum function of all the systems in your body as well as their ability to communicate with each other properly....Minimizing the stress on your body, both inside and out, is the way to keep your body happy and healthy."

Life is a journey with many destinations along the way. As you travel down the winding path of life, your health will be a key factor in determining your ability to enjoy every aspect of your journey. Your health defines the boundaries, or sides, of the path. When you stray from the path your ability to move along your life's journey becomes more difficult. Your body will let you know when you are pushing the boundaries of the path by presenting symptoms to alert you that you are moving off the path. The path to health defines the direction you will move along life's journey. Your health is the key to a more successful life.

Your health is much more than not feeling sick or tired. Health is the optimum function of all the systems in your body as well as their ability to communicate with each other properly. Although I will break down your body into easily identifiable systems to describe how to maintain your health, you must remember that they also have to work together and communicate with each other. Every part of your body is important when you are considering your health. Your body can not stay healthy without constant communication between all systems in your body. As we discuss the different systems of your body and how to care for them, we will also talk about the ways that they affect your overall health, as well as the health of other systems. We will start with connecting the outside or physical body to the inside systems along with how to maintain your physical condition.

The big picture:

Minimizing the stress on your body, both inside and out, is the way to keep your body happy and healthy. Keeping stress levels low is the key to maintaining our physical condition, especially when it comes to the health of our bones. For example, stress will cause an elevation in the output of cortisol by our adrenal glands. A prolonged elevation of cortisol will predispose us to osteoporosis and weaken our bones. In other words, you must minimize the stress on your body to keep your bones healthy. Please see

Figure 7 for a list of common and major stressors on the body.

Not only do the adrenal glands help regulate stress and the body's ability to adapt to stress, they also regulate our energy levels by producing hormones. They make precursors to the major "sex" hormones in our body: estrogen, testosterone, and progesterone. The "sex" hormones play a major role in managing our energy levels, as well as helping us manage the expression of our mood. Keeping your stressors minimized will help prevent hormone imbalances in your body. See *Figure 8* for some common signs and symptoms to watch out for, which may be due to chronic stress and its effect on the adrenal glands.

Figure 7- *Common and Major Stressors*

Frequent and/or extreme fluctuations in our Blood Sugar	Allowing our body to get too hot or too cold (extreme weather conditions)
Over-training	Emotional stress
Food Sensitivities	Pharmaceutical drugs
Synthetic vitamins and supplements	Not eating food with proper nutrient levels
Autoimmunity	Infection
Environmental chemicals, like BPA, pesticides, herbicides, smog, heavy metals	Conventional Dental work, especially mercury amalgam fillings and root canals
Recreational drugs, such as alcohol, tobacco	Dysbiosis & sub-clinical infections

Figure 8- *Common Signs of Stress*

Weight gain in the abdomen	High blood pressure
Depression	Anxiety
Insomnia	Waking up tired
Fatigue	Feeling worn down
Osteoporosis	Dysmenorrhea
Infertility	Loss of sex drive
Getting sick frequently	Low immune system
Memory lapses	Low learning abilities
Pain that won't go away	Mood Swings

Caring for your muscles:

Physical fitness starts on the inside. If you nourish your body properly, then fitness can be obtained relatively easily, and happily. When you minimize the stress on your body, you allow your body's metabolism to work as intended. Our body is designed to favor fat burning. Increased fat on our body is a sign that our body is stressed and is not working as designed. The first step in physical fitness should always be to minimize stress.

If you have not exercised for an extended period of time or if you have never exercised, prepare the inside of your body first, then move on toward exercising the physical body. If you are currently exercising regularly and want to improve your health, take a step back to assess how your exercise program is affecting your health. Are you stressing your body by <u>over</u> training?

A word of caution prior to changing your workout protocols. Please consult your health care professional of choice, prior to starting any exercise routine, to make sure your body will be able to handle the rigor of the changes.

Now, consider these two questions when deciding how much to exercise: What has your physical activity been like over the last 6 months? Have you ever exercised?

The answers to those questions will give you your starting point. If you have never *really* exercised, then don't start now, at least not until you have prepared the inside of your body. Go back to the

How To Eat And Drink section of this manual and begin by following those guidelines for 30 days prior to beginning your exercise program (See *Figures 1, 2, 3*). This is especially important if you are or were a smoker. When you start a new exercise regimen, the demand on your nervous system and energy production system (think about your blood sugar) will have to be ready to meet the new demands that you are putting on them. For most people, these systems are usually not prepared to keep up with their new exercise demands and the exercise ends up being more stressful than helpful. In other words, your muscles, ligaments, and bones (musculoskeletal system) may be prepared for a day of exercise, but your nervous system and energy production systems will usually not be able to keep up. This will leave you sore, achy, increase your risk of injury, increase your risk for cardiovascular accidents (strokes and heart attacks), and lengthen your recovery time.

With that in mind, **everyday** should begin with a short burst of physical activity. This activity should be performed long enough to increase your *heart rate***(see note at the end of this paragraph)* to double its resting rate in the morning (1-2 minutes for those that have not exercised within the past 6 months, or have never exercised, and then increase it slowly according to your fitness level). The activation of your heart and muscle tissues will help regulate your body's energy production and get your metabolism going by stimulating your adrenal glands. These are small glands that sit on top of our kidneys. Just like we have two kidneys, one on each side of our body, we have two adrenal glands. These glands help to regulate our body's ability to manage stress, electrolytes (salts, acids, and bases), and hormone production. The adrenal glands are predominantly regulated by our nervous system (brain and nerves), and they operate in rhythmic cycles unless we become stressed. These rhythmic cycles help coordinate our energy level throughout the day, as well as, our sleep cycles at night. That is the reason why morning exercise is important, it helps accentuate the natural rhythm of our energy production cycles. The key to maintaining our physical condition is to keep the inside of our body happy. This means minimizing all stressors in our life.

*** *To measure your heart rate, locate your radial pulse or carotid pulse. The radial pulse can be found by pressing lightly on the thumb side of your wrist, just beneath the palm, on inside of the bone that connects the wrist to the root of the thumb. The carotid pulse can be found by touching the bone behind either ear and then sliding your fingers along the jaw line toward the side of your throat and applying light pressure into your neck. Once you've found your pulse, count the number of pulsations or beats over one minute. This is your resting heart rate in beats per minute. Optionally, you can count the number of pulsations or beats over 15 seconds and multiply it by 4 to estimate your heart rate in beats per minute (bpm).*

Instead of getting on the treadmill, or doing "cardio" for an hour before your workout, you should: Start each day with at least 2-5 minutes of exercise to get the heart rate up to double its resting rate, (but no more than 30 minutes of exercise, because you need to eat). Eat a good breakfast with a strong protein component. Strength train sometime throughout the day (10-30 minutes depending upon your ability). Strength training will encourage stronger bones and muscles in your body.

For beginners, or those that have not had a regular exercise routine for the last six months, your physical body will not likely be the limiting factor in your ability to endure the workout described above. It will typically be your nervous system and other internal organs ability to adapt to the stress of exercise. Therefore, I want to remind you to start with exercising good health on the inside of your body first. Second, add the morning exercise. Third, add the strength training. Then fourth, add the "cardio" exercises to build endurance. This is a recipe for successful, healthy body function. The topics of professional strength and endurance training are beyond the scope of this basic manual. Exercise caution in your choices, and remember that over-training is a stress on your body, so push yourself responsibly!

Caring for your Brain and nervous system:

Your nervous system needs two things to survive and thrive: activation and fuel! Activation comes from the stimulation of our nervous system by moving through the world around us and interpreting our interactions with it, as well as the production and use of neurotransmitters. Neurotransmitters are the signals that our body uses to send messages through our nervous system. Repetitive stimulation, whether it is opening our eyes everyday and looking around at the different colors, shapes, and lights, or learning to write our name, activates our nervous system and helps keep it healthy. The adequate production and use of neurotransmitters allows us to feel happiness and joy, complete tasks, not feel anxious, and remember information. These two systems of activation are essential to the health of our brain, as well as the health of our nervous system.

Fuel to fire our nervous system comes, primarily, from oxygen and glucose. We breathe in oxygen and it is carried throughout our body by our blood. Our blood not only carries oxygen, but also the glucose we get from our food. These two fuels drive our nervous system's function. Our brain does not have the ability to store oxygen and glucose, so it is our job to maintain the constant availability of the right amounts of these fuels. To take care of our brain and nerves, we need to manage these four things:

- Nervous System Stimulation
- Neurotransmitters
- Oxygen
- Glucose

If you take the time each day to follow the physical fitness recommendations and eating guidelines we discussed earlier, nourishing your nervous system with stimulation will be easier. (Please recall the sections: *Maintaining Your Health* and subsection *Caring For Your Muscles* as well as *Figures 1,2,3*) Take 30 minutes each day to work on a hobby that does not involve the use of electronics. This will help minimize your stress, and give you the opportunity to nourish your nervous system. Make sure you have at least three hobbies to rotate into your daily routine so that you exercise different parts of your brain. You should pick hobbies that improve or practice one or more of the following types of activities: Accuracy, Balance, Rhythm/Timing, or Eye Movements. Some activities that improve **accuracy** are: playing a musical instrument, throwing darts, sewing, shooting baskets, or painting/drawing. **Balance** is improved with activities such as riding a bike, surfing, skateboarding, skiing, yoga, or tai chi. **Rhythm/Timing** activities include: playing music, clapping to the beat of a song, playing catch, juggling, or dancing. Exercises and activities that involve **eye movements** are: racquetball, yoga while maintaining focus on a fixed or stationary target during poses, driving, or sightseeing.

Proper production of neurotransmitters is dependent upon maintaining the healthy eating habits we discussed before (See the **Basic Rules of Eating** and **Figures 1, 2, 3**). Imbalances in your blood sugar levels will decrease your body's ability to produce key neurotransmitters (Refer to **Figures 4, 5**). This can lead toward the symptoms of depression, as well as emotional instability, and decreased memory capabilities. In addition, not eating food containing adequate amounts of essential fatty acids will affect the production of neurotransmitters, and can lead toward anxiety, or anxious feelings. The availability and use of essential fatty acids can also be depleted from eating trans fats, partially hydrogenated oils, and/or hydrogenated oils, which can lead to similar symptoms of anxiety. Remember that all of the cells in your body maintain a wall around them made of fatty acids, along with cholesterol and proteins throughout the wall. Cholesterol is also the building block of several key hormones in your body. You need cholesterol to survive, just not the wrong sources. Here are some great sources of *essential fatty acids (EFA's): fish with a low mercury content, avocado, olive oil, coconut oil, and raw tree nuts.*

Caring for your Digestive organs:

When we bring food into our body for nourishment, we must break it down into small pieces so that it may be absorbed into our body. This process starts with chewing. We must chew our food for three major reasons. First, chewing physically breaks our food into smaller pieces. Second, our saliva contains components that help to begin the breakdown of the molecular components of our food so that they may pass into our body for nourishment. Third, it begins to activate the parts of our nervous system that regulate digestion. While the food is in our mouth we can also taste the flavor of the food. This sense of flavor, or taste, allows our brain to know exactly what is coming into our digestive system, so that it can coordinate the digestion of the food. This is activation of our nervous system on a basic level, and it helps keep our nervous system healthy. It also underscores the point that all systems of your body are in constant communication all at once. The health of one body system will have a beneficial or detrimental influence on the health of your other systems.

As the food moves down into our stomach, our nervous system will coordinate the movement of more blood to the digestive system so nutrients may be absorbed and transported. This does not happen efficiently during times of stress. When the body is stressed, our nervous system will send more resources toward our musculoskeletal system and away from our digestive system. To keep your digestive system in good working order we must minimize our stress. The presence of proper amounts of digestive acids and enzymes, along with the proper digestive pH level are essential components to normal digestion in the stomach and down the rest of the digestive tract. Stress on your body over long periods of time will hinder the digestive process by inhibiting the ability of the body to regulate the pH of your digestive tract. We use the pH scale to measure the acidity of a fluid or other area of the body. It is a measurement scale that accounts for the number of hydrogen ions present in a fluid or area of the body. This scale is one of many tools that help us understand when changes have been made in your body's overall ability to maintain health, or to properly digest.

The food in the stomach must be broken down adequately before it is moved into the small intestine, or this can increase stress on your body. Once the food is in the small intestine, the rhythm of digestion continues to progress and the food will interact with more enzymes and the pH is adjusted to optimize further breakdown of your food. More digestion will occur along the length of the small intestine, as well as absorption of nutrients. The remnants of the digested food will continue through to the large intestine passing through the ileocecal valve, which mechanically helps prevent back flow from the large intestine into the small intestine. Your appendix helps regulate inflammation and address irritation at this important juncture of your intestines. *(A history of appendicitis or appendectomy may be your first clue that you have sensitivities to staple foods in your diet.)* Along the entire length of the intestines, both large and small, are symbiotic bacteria and other microorganisms collectively referred to as your intestinal flora (for simplicity I am going to refer to the intestinal flora as bacteria, but it should be understood that your intestinal flora is comprised of more than just bacteria). When they are present in the right balance, these bacteria will help with further breakdown of your food, as well as the production of nutrients that we are not able to produce without the presence of these bacteria. When our body is bombarded with stress on a consistent basis, these bacteria can move out of balance. Bacteria that are not meant to be the predominant bacteria in our intestines will be allowed to dominate our intestinal tract. This change in bacterial growth may present itself as an infection, or a dysbiosis. A dysbiosis refers to either an overgrowth or suppression of the growth of microorganisms in our intestinal flora. A dysbiosis does not necessarily have an acute infectious symptom (such as fever or diarrhea). To maintain the health of our digestive system we must minimize the stress on our body. This includes physical, chemical, energetic, and emotional stress.

Many of us are educated about the individual roles of different organ systems in our body, but most of us are not taught about the intricate interplay between all systems of our body. The relationship between different organs in our body allows us the opportunity to correct problems before they cause disease. We just need to learn how to interpret the calls for help before they become too loud to ignore. For example, you may think: "Well, how does going outside all winter long without proper protective clothing affect my digestion?" Or. "How does over-training have an influence on my immune system?" They are indirectly related because they affect parts of the same body. Different parts that are in constant communication with every other part of your body. **Any stressor** that we have mentioned (see *Figures 7, 8*), and some that may not even be on the list in this book, may have an impact on your body and will indirectly influence all systems of our body! If you understand that point, and put into action a total stress relief plan, you will have taken a large part of your health back into your own hands. Proper digestive health can be maintained by following the healthy eating habits we discussed earlier (See the **Basic Rules of Eating** and **Figures 1, 2, 3**). Stress from imbalances in your blood sugar levels is the most common and one of the greatest stressors on your body. Eating habits that favor stability of your blood sugar (Refer to **Figures 4, 5**) are essential to maintaining digestive health. Additionally, your diet should include ample amounts of fermented foods. These foods will encourage stabilization of the intestinal flora during times of stress, as well as during your recovery from the effects of stress. *Fermented foods should be consumed at each major meal and different varieties should be rotated throughout the day.* For example: you may have a fermented coconut product with your breakfast (like raw, unpasteurized coconut yogurt), kombucha tea with your lunch, and sauerkraut with your dinner. Three different varieties of fermented foods at each of your three major meals.

Caring for your Reproductive Organs and Hormone Producing Glands:

The reproductive system in our body is one of the greatest examples of how our system is intricately connected. Our reproductive system is constantly on alert to do its job, even though we are not constantly trying to reproduce. So, when looking at our reproductive system, we must consider the larger hormonal systems of our body. This includes all organs that create and influence hormone production.

What do hormones do? In general, our hormones are chemical signals produced by an organ that are designed to have an influence on other organs or systems. These hormones, in large part, are designed to manage and regulate our functional energy levels. I think of the hormones as our body's way of bridging the gap between molecular energy (the energy that powers the cells in our body) and the energy of larger body structures. They function as a means to regulate our use of energy that comes from outside the body into usable energy inside our body. This energy can then be used to drive the functional interaction between our body and the rest of the world. The hormone systems are greatly influenced by the availability of nutrients from our food. Imbalances in this system are the direct result of what we eat, drink, and breathe in. Physical and emotional stress will also greatly impact our hormone production along with our body's regulation of their numbers. It is these hormone systems that cause the indirect communication between the different systems of our body and allow one system to interact with the rest. They connect our body into one functional unit. In essence, they make you, YOU!

The ability of our reproductive system and other hormone producing glands to function properly, as well as stay healthy, is dependent upon maintaining the healthy eating habits we discussed before (See the **Basic Rules of Eating** and **Figures 1, 2, 3**). Fluctuations in your blood sugar levels will decrease your body's ability to produce, transport, and use hormones efficiently and effectively (Refer to *Figures 4, 5*). To further facilitate the function of the reproductive system we must establish a total stress relief plan, that includes reduction of physical, chemical, energetic, and emotional stress (Reference *Figures 7 & 8)*.

The guidelines that we have covered thus far in the manual are related to the general health of your body. If you view those guidelines as the boundaries of a path leading to health, you will see that staying on this path, or returning to this path will lead you toward health. There are several organs and physiological systems of the body that contribute to your health that have not been covered in this basic manual. That is done with the intent of making sure that you can easily read through this manual and immediately have the basic information necessary for maintaining and improving your health. The guidelines in this manual are the foundation to building the health of your body.

GETTING YOUR HEALTH BACK

"Most chronic conditions that affect our society are largely due to lifestyle choices that cause people to stray away from the path of health... Follow the recipe for success as laid out in this manual and you can start to take the steps toward getting your life back!"

Recovery From Pain

What is pain exactly? Pain signals are sent to the emotional center of our brain. This is why you may have heard it said: "pain is an emotion." Here are some more inherent rules in regard to pain:

The perception of pain can be increased by having a diet poor in beneficial fats, and/or heavy in unhealthy fats.

Chronic pain actually improves your body's ability to register pain...you can get good at being in pain. This means that you will feel pain more often than you should.

Poor health of the nervous system can (and often does) sabotage your body's natural ability to decrease pain. Poor health of the nervous system can be the sole cause of your pain.

Pain is inhibited by movement. Think about your reaction to getting your finger smashed...you shake it!

Just as we discussed previously, all systems of our body are intricately connected and have an influence on each other. The same is true of physical pain. Let's use the example of a sprained ankle. What caused you to sprain your ankle and have pain? Was it that you were trying to change directions while you were walking, or running, and your ankle was not strong enough to support you? Were you under some sort of stress when it happened? Were you playing a sport, or maybe, just had something on your mind while performing a routine activity? Why was it, that this time, you were injured?

Most of us (especially doctors, of all types) are taught to disconnect the different systems of our body, and treat the physical body as a separate entity. We think that an ankle sprain is merely caused by a weak ankle, taking a "bad" step, landing "wrong", tripping, etc. That logic could not be more flawed. Consider the ankle injury scenario we discussed earlier. What if that person had a tendency to eat the Standard American Diet (S.A.D.). An all-American who ate all-American food, like: spaghetti and meatballs, hamburgers, hotdogs, or coffee and donuts for breakfast. The day of that ankle injury could have been just like any other day in their life: Juice and a bagel for breakfast at church, followed by a trip to the gym to get some exercise.

The interplay between this person and their environment could be looked at this way: This person took the time to nourish their spirit and body by going to church and the gym, however, the bagel and juice for breakfast have done a few things to undermine their success. If this is their typical breakfast, think about what it is doing to the "fire" inside their body. Both the juice and bagel are turned into large amounts of energy in the body, or in other words they raise the blood sugar very quickly and provide a quick burst of energy. However, this energy will be used up very quickly, like burning a piece of paper in a fire. (Think about how paper burns as opposed to wood. The paper will burn quickly and brightly, and then be gone. The wood will burn steadily over a longer period of time.) This spike in blood sugar will inevitably be followed by a drop in blood sugar. Once the energy is used up and there is no more food coming in, their body will initiate a stress response to stabilize the blood sugar and their energy level. This will cause stress in their body.

Is this stress enough to allow for an injury of the ankle to occur? How could that happen? The physical body is just one system that is in constant communication with all other systems of our body. If the spike in blood sugar was followed by an insulin surge and a rise in cortisol output from the adrenal glands, it could set the stage for instability of the muscular and ligamentous structures of the ankle. Ligament laxity caused by an increase in cortisol output by the adrenal glands, followed by landing "wrong" on your ankle will have direct impact on the severity of your ankle injury. When you look at the body as an interconnected entity, you can see that: stress in one part of our body (when compounded by stress in other parts of the body) will increase our overall stress level. This will cause a decrease in our ability to handle all of our total stress load over an extended period of time and can set the stage for injury.

Let's say that instead of an ankle sprain, that was caused by you doing something, that you were lying down on the ground and your spouse stepped on your ankle. Does interplay between the different systems of my body have an influence on my recovery? Does that interplay have an influence on the severity of my injury? If you had a passive role in the trauma, your body's ability to withstand that trauma is still dependent on the pre-existing condition of your body. Obviously, if the trauma were more severe, like a car rolling over your ankle, there must be a breaking point for what your body can take. In either case, your body's ability to recover will be dependent upon the overall stress level inside your body. Your experience of pain will be determined by how severe the damage is, multiplied by your body's ability to cope with pain. This is determined by your diet in combination with the other stressors on your body.

A good rule of thumb is that you should recover from most injuries in 4-6 weeks. If you do not, there is typically something going on that is perpetuating the problem from the inside. This can be inappropriate signals in or from your nervous system, or the effects of stress on the inside of your body. Pain is temporary, when it persists your body is asking you for help.

If you have chronic pain (*in general pain that has not improved after 6-8 weeks or lasts longer than 12 weeks*), you should seek the help of a qualified healthcare practitioner. However, there are some things you can do on your own to help. The most common cause of perpetual, chronic pain in the body is the cumulative effect of all your stressors. When you are injured, you must not only minimize your stressors, but do your best to eliminate all of them until you have fully recovered. This can include: correcting any underlying abnormalities in you blood sugar, eating increased amounts of essential fatty acids (EFA's), and exercises to ensure optimum activation of your brain. (Please refer to the ***Basic Rules of Eating*** and

Figures 1, 2, 3, 7 & 8) Your doctor should know how to help you with some, or all of these. If not, you should reassess your relationship with your doctor and/or add another doctor to your care team. When you take the stressors away from your body, your body will take care of you.

Please Note- In the absence of trauma, your pain is usually caused by or promoted by internal dysfunction.

Dealing with Digestive Problems:

Many people compare their symptoms to other people's symptoms to assess whether or not what they are experiencing is normal. This is no longer an acceptable way to determine healthy digestive status. The new "normal person" today is not healthy. Comparing yourself to "normal" will often times lead you down a path away from optimal health. *So, what should I do?* Compare yourself to someone who does not have any symptoms. Which means, if you have digestive symptoms you are not digesting normally. The "experts" in the health field who would tell you, "Well, you are just getting older," or "that's normal for someone your age," are not the people you should be listening to. They need to be re-educated, because most of the time they are telling you the wrong information. It would be more accurate if they said, "I don't know what's causing your symptoms," or "try seeing a doctor of chiropractic, naturopathic doctor, holistic MD, or an acupuncturist, I don't know what is wrong with you." Our healthcare system is great for acute (things that are hurting or injured right now) care for the digestive system, but when you consistently use acute therapies as a long term solution, you are not going to keep anyone healthy. You need to focus on what is causing the stress on your body and resulting in digestive dysfunction. If you have a digestive problem you need to look very closely at what initiates the digestive process, THE FOOD AND DRINK THAT YOU PUT IN YOUR MOUTH! It is far too common for people with digestive problems to hear that what they eat does not matter, and that could not be farther from the truth.

To illustrate the effect of our food on our body, let's look at an extreme example: consider someone who has a severe allergic reaction to peanuts. So severe, that they will have an anaphylactic reaction, break out into hives, and their throat will swell shut. Would it make sense to give them a limitless supply of self-injecting epinephrine shots, tell them "Don't worry about eating peanuts just take your shots to clear up your reaction, you will be fine". Or, would it make sense to educate the person on their reaction and teach them how to avoid exposure to peanuts, as well as how to use the epinephrine in case of an accidental exposure. Of course, the second scenario makes more sense, and that is actually the way a peanut allergy is cared for medically. The logic that drives that model of care seems to disappear when it comes to less life-threatening conditions, such as constipation, heartburn, irritable bowels, GERD, Crohn's Disease, IBD, etc. Instead, people are often given remedies that take care of the symptoms but do not identify the cause of the problems. It was not always this way, but with the ever growing influence of the pharmaceutical companies on medical care and public perception, we can see that most doctors are valued for the drugs and relief they can give you, not for what that doctor can teach you about how to take care of yourself. The sad truth is that there are far too many doctors and patients who are content with that dynamic. When it comes to our digestive health, too many healthcare professionals are lost in a lost world. The good news is that you can empower yourself to improve your health. When you take care of your body it will take care of you. Remember, if you have a digestive problem your diet should be the first place you look for answers, and prolonged use of acute therapies should be the last.

Why should I be concerned over a little upset stomach when I eat? It's normal, right? This line of thinking is destroying the health of upwards of 40% of the population in the US. That 40% represents an estimate of the number of Americans who have a food sensitivity, whether diagnosed or not, that is causing stress and inflammation in their body.

This number is expected to continue to grow and is why the gluten-free fad has continued to gain momentum *(Remember just because a food is labeled gluten-free, organic, or vegan does not mean that it is a quality food. There is a lot of junk food that carries those labels.)*. The idea that food sensitivities only affect our digestive system is an obsolete concept. Consider that only 1 in 8 people who have celiac disease have digestive symptoms as their primary complaint. (Celiac disease is one of the most common lifelong diseases affecting Americans, in which your body's immune system attacks and destroys your intestinal walls.) The other 7 out of 8 people with celiac disease have no obvious digestive symptoms. Great, right? No, those 7 people die sooner and have more debilitating sickness than those with digestive symptoms. The reason, is they never relate what they are eating to their problem and are often not diagnosed for many years. This is because their symptoms are unrelated to their digestive system and their doctors cannot connect the dots. What is the trigger in celiac disease? It is one of the proteins in wheat, gluten! Which means, every time they eat wheat products (bread, pastries, most salad dressings, soup, etc) their body will attack and destroy intestinal tissue.

It is becoming increasingly apparent in the research community that what we eat has a wide-reaching effect on how we feel, as well as the status of our health. It may still take some time (hopefully within the next 5-10 years) before it becomes a mainstream concept that once again you are what you eat. In short, the most common food sensitivities that should be considered as potential stressors are grains (especially gluten containing grains: wheat, rye, barley, etc.), dairy, soy and corn. Food sensitivities are one of the primary culprits in causing digestive symptoms.

So, what do you do when things go wrong in the digestive system? **First**, you go back to a basic diet (See the ***Basic Rules of Eating***). Please refer to ***Figures 1, 2 & 3.*** Follow the dietary guidelines in this book very strictly. **Second**, you must take an inventory of your current stressors. See ***Figures 7 & 8*** and make a list of your stressors. Look over the list and take care of what you can on your own and seek help for the rest. Start to eat food that will nourish your body, and drink the appropriate amount of water. This will often eliminate more than 50% of your problems, for most people. This is because your basic diet (described earlier) will eliminate common allergens. If you have any doubt about which other stressor should be addressed first, keep this in mind, you must get fuel to your nervous system. Do you have anemia, or a blood sugar abnormality? If you haven't been checked for this, you should strongly consider it. What is the status of your intestines? Do you get bloated? If you have intestinal-type symptoms you should be screened for food sensitivities and possibly look into a stool microbial profile to check the status of your intestinal flora, at the very least. Are you constantly stressed? Find some time for yourself EVERYDAY where you just relax, and nothing else.

Dealing with Low or No Energy:

Do you feel run down, a lack of energy, fatigue, or are you tired all of the time? Why? This is your body's signal that your energy requirements for managing your stressors, along with your everyday functions, have not been met for an extended period of time. This means that you are causing your body stress by having continued, or prolonged stress that your body no longer has the capacity to deal with. The result causes changes in your body's ability to regulate it's energy rhythms. The most basic requirements to keep our body and nervous system from being stressed are to provide proper availability of glucose, oxygen, stimulation, and neurotransmitters. When you have active stressors for extended periods of time the availability of those basic requirements decreases, and the result is a change in your energy level, recovery time, and/or vitality. How do you fix this? You must start to provide the proper availability of glucose, oxygen, stimulation, and neurotransmitters to your body, along with minimizing or eliminating your stressors.

Go back to the basics, to care for your body. You must eat and drink to nourish your body. Please refer to the **Basic Rules of Eating** and **Figures 1, 2, 3.** This will alleviate any stressors related to your blood sugar, or the availability of glucose, and help provide the building blocks for your neurotransmitters and hormones. You must care for your physical condition. Begin each day with exercise, to help reset your natural energy rhythm. Strength training, along with dedicating 20 minutes each day to a hobby as described earlier (refer to **Maintaining Your Health**, the subsection titled **Brain and nervous system**) , and taking two 10 minute relaxation breaks (where you do nothing but rest your mind and breathe, but no other activity for your mind or body) to stimulate, oxygenate, and unwind your nervous system. Then you must go through the list of stressors one by one, and begin to eliminate as many as you can. Please refer to **Figures 7 & 8.** After that, go through the list again and remove one more. You must remove these stressors to give your body a chance to heal. Care for your body's energy systems like you would anything else that breaks in your body. Please refer to **Figures 4 & 5** for symptoms related to your blood sugar. Think of it like this: If you broke the long bone of your thigh (the femur), would you continue to walk on it? The pain and damage would be constant reminders that you were not allowing your body to heal from the trauma that caused the problem. When you feel run down, have no energy, are fatigued, or are tired all of the time, the ability of your body to provide rhythmic availability of energy has been injured, or broken. Those symptoms are your body's call for help, just like pain with a broken bone. You must nurture these systems back to health with the same care you would a broken bone...a minimum of 6-8 weeks of careful nurturing. If you do this, you will improve your health. It is always best to consult a holistic healthcare professional properly trained in evaluating what level of health you are in, or if not available, consult a general healthcare practitioner to make sure you have not already progressed to the point of disease.

My doctor told me I have_____, now what?

"There is a zebra in your bathtub, and he is eating and eliminating you out of house and home and

generally making your life miserable. Someone comes to visit your home, recognizes the disruption of normal activity, and tells you that the zebra's name is "Charley." Then you feel much better, at least at first. However, the awareness of his name does nothing to solve the fact that there is an offensive zebra in your bathtub who is eating and eliminating you out of your domicile. What IS important is "How do I get the zebra out of my bathtub", and secondly, "How did he get there in the first place so I can keep it from happening again!"

Giving the zebra a name is like a doctor giving a patient a diagnosis. This is fine as long as the "diagnosis" is not the only goal of the clinician. Diagnostics should be therapy oriented rather than an academic exercise. There must be a therapeutic course implied by a diagnosis. In certain acute illnesses (e.g., pneumonia, appendicitis) the diagnosis directs the therapy. In chronic conditions, including most of those processes associated with aging, the diagnosis serves little purpose in directing corrective or preventive therapy."

Excerpt from Diagnosing the process, not just the name by Dr. Walter H. Schmitt, expanding on a parable used by the late, great, Dr. George Goodheart.

Most chronic conditions that affect our society are largely due to lifestyle choices that cause people to stray away from the path laid out in this manual of health. The zebra in the story above gets into the house because the house was not cared for properly and became compromised. Not following the guidelines of this manual, is like not caring for your house properly. Your house (or your body) will then be susceptible to intrusion by the zebra (or you will be susceptible to the development of a disease). Respect for your body's condition is of the utmost importance. The chronic nature of most diseases should not water down the acute effects they can have on your body. That means that the immediate or severe symptoms due to your disease should be managed quickly. In addition, you should follow the advice of your treating doctor in the management of your disease to ensure that it does not cause any permanent damage. However, that does not mean that you must stand by your doctor if they are unwilling to work with you on your quest toward health. Don't be afraid to seek the opinion of another doctor, preferably one with additional holistic education. But, remember, it is ultimately your responsibility to take care of yourself, and you will have to do the work to restore your health. It cannot be done for you. Your doctor's job is to facilitate your recovery, but you and your body are going to have to do the work.

Open your mind to the needs of your body and the effects of chronic stressors. As you do, you will begin to see exactly how going back to the basic nurturing of your body will change the way you feel. Take your medication, have any necessary surgery, follow your supplement prescription, but nurture your body before, during, and after to ensure that you can do your best to heal.

Follow the recipe for success as laid out in this manual and you can start to take the steps toward getting your life back! Be advised that once your body has not been nourished for an extended period of time you run the risk of losing your health. Then once your health is lost, becoming sick, or the development of a named condition (disease) is usually just a matter of time. This means that your body has been deeply injured and you should nourish it for a minimum of six months with great care to eliminate all stressors. Please reference the **Basic Rules of Eating**, the subsection titled **Water** and **Figures 1, 2, 3, 4, 5, 6, 7, & 8.** It can take upwards of 24 months of nurturing without the aid of a properly trained healthcare professional, dependent upon the severity of your condition. Without the guidance of a properly trained healthcare professional, you may also find limitations to your successful recovery. If you have not noticed recovery after nourishing your body and eliminating your stressors within 3-6 months, or if they plateau during that period, you should seek help from a healthcare professional trained in evaluating optimum health and add him/her to your healthcare team. Do not be afraid to help yourself, or ask for help when you need it. It is important to be able to trust your health advisers, so that your recovery is as quick as possible.

When all else fails, dealing with a heavy diagnosis:

This is the stage of health where all seems lost, and sometimes can be. All of us will be here at some point in our life, but this is where none of us want to be. You can be stuck here at the brink of death and dysfunction and feel there is no hope, or you may have the advanced stages of disease and your doctors may have told you that you only have x number of days, months, or years to live. This stage is one and the same for most doctors, despite a huge difference in the capacity of the patient to live when they're told they will die, or to get their health back when they're told they can only be sick. You can be in this stage before your time, and stay here for many years, or this can be a transition stage that is passed through quickly and with serenity. Your state of health may be the determining factor. Whatever the case may be, when all else fails, and you feel like this is it, what do you do?

To change your situation at this point, you must understand the message in this manual: YOU MUST CHANGE YOUR LIFE. From this point, and going forward, you cannot go back to the way you were attempting to nourish your body. You must be forever changed. The basic eating and drinking recommendations we have discussed should be your new, normal habits. Please refer to the **Basic Rules of Eating**, the subsection titled **Water** and **Figures 1, 2, 3, 4, 5, & 6.** You must find a holistic healthcare practitioner to add to your team, to help you find the right path of how to eat, drink, and live with as few stressors as possible, as quickly as possible. Please refer to **Figures 7 & 8** to aid in your identification of your particular stressors. To get the most out of your life (not just years of living, but the best possible years of living), your new normal habits must be healthy and nourishing for your body. Your job, more than ever, is to help re-establish nourishment for your body on a daily basis. This manual is only as good as your ability to use it with committed dedication.

To make this change you must adhere to three rules:

1. **You must be ready, willing, and able to make a diet and lifestyle change and commit to it.**

2. **You have to take personal responsibility for your health.** It is your body, and you must care for it!

3. **You have to be willing to make a personal investment in your health.** Improving your health will take time, so you must be able to commit your time to taking care of yourself. Your insurance typically will not pay for help that is geared toward improving your health, so you may have to invest financially in care that will focus on your health, not merely eliminating or preventing disease.

If you or a loved one is suffering, and are in need of help, here are the criterion for selecting a healthcare professional to help you:

You must trust that person. They will have your health in their hands, and you must trust their leadership.

You must fulfill your end of the treatments. Most of the time, recovering your health requires more work from you than your doctor. If you cannot do your part, how will they do theirs? It is your right to ask for an explanation from your doctor if your recovery is not going on schedule. You should know why you are doing what you're doing. It will make you work harder to keep up with your end of the treatment. Get a second opinion if you are not making progress.

You, and your doctor, both have to be able to recognize when you need help from your doctor or when you must help yourself. If you need to work harder, they must be willing to let you know and you must trust them enough to listen.

They should be in good health themselves, or actively making an effort to improve their health. They must walk the walk.

Why have I never heard of these simple life lessons? You may have heard some, or all of what you have read in this manual. However, this is the first time that it has been laid out in front of you along with a common sense rationale of why you should follow the path to health. The truth is, that we all have an idea of what it takes to be healthy, we just need to listen to that part of us without the static of today's world drowning out the message.

You can take it from here.

In Good Health,

Dr. Richard L. Robles, DC

APPENDIX

This appendix contains the information necessary to follow your path to health. If you need a quick reference this is the place for you.

Basic Rules of Eating:

Eat food that has not been changed from the way that it looked when it was walking around, or living in the ground.

1. *Eat breakfast or a morning snack within 30 minutes of waking up in the morning.*

2. *Each of your three main meals should contain vegetables and a protein source, with snacking occurring throughout the day (at least one snack in between each meal).*

3. *Vegetables should be eaten in quantities that are equal to twice your intake of fruit. This does not mean to eat less fruit, in general, it means to <u>eat more vegetables</u>.*

Water:

The first basic formula:
Drink 1 quart of water for every 50 lbs of body weight.

The second basic formula:
Body weight divided in half equals the number of ounces you should drink.

Your optimal water intake is usually in between the calculations from these two formulas (Remember 1 quart equals 32 ounces, and 1 gallon equals 4 quarts or 128 ounces).

Figure 1- *The four basic food groups*

Group 1	Group 2	Group 3	Group 4
Wild food sources, from a unpolluted environment	Organic Meat, Eggs, Vegetables, & Fruit	Conventional Meat, Vegetables, & Fruit	Processed Food
			Organic Tea
Organic Sustainably-Raised Vegetables, & Fruit	Fermented Conventional Foods	Organic Grains	Organic Coffee
		Organic Processed Food	Organic Sweeteners
Fermented Organic Foods	Organic nuts, beans, lentils, legumes	Farm-raised fish	Grains
Organic pasture-raised Meats & Eggs			
Wild-caught fish			

**Note: Organic coffee, tea, and sweeteners have been included in Group 4 due to the stimulatory effect of these items.

Figure 2- *How much to eat of each food group*

	People with a heavy diagnosis	People diagnosed with a disease	People with Daily symptoms	No Daily Symptoms
Group 1	85%	80%	75%	70%
Group 2	15%	15%	23%	20%
Group 3	0%	5%	5%	5%
Group 4	0%	0%	2%	5%

**Note- *Another way to look at this chart is as follows: 70% means that 7 out of every 10 items you eat will come from Group 1, 20% means that 2 out of every 10 items you eat will come from Group 2, 5% means that 1 out of every 20 items you eat will come from Group 3, 5% means that 1 out of every 20 items you eat will come from Group 4 for individuals with no daily symptoms. Therefore, most of the food you eat should come from groups 1 and 2 and very little should come from groups 3 and 4.*

Figure 3- *Different types of Foods by category*

Animal Meat	Fish, eggs, beef, turkey, shellfish, chicken, game meats
Vegetables	Asparagus, artichoke, broccoli, cabbage, carrots, celery, collard greens, dandelion greens, garlic, kale, kohlrabi, leeks, lettuce, mustard greens, onions, parsley, potatoes, radish, rhubarb, rutabaga, salads, shallots, spinach, squash, sweet potatoes, turnips, water chestnuts, watercress, yams, zucchini
Fruit	Fresh apples, apricots, avocados, berries, cherries, grapefruit, grapes, lemons, oranges, peaches, pears, plums, nectarines, prunes, mango, melons, pineapple
Fermented Foods	Sauerkraut, kombucha, fermented coconut products, kimchi, fermented vegetables & fruit
Herbs and Spices	Anise, basil, bay leaf, black pepper, cilantro, coriander, cumin, garlic, ginger, lemongrass, mint, onion, oregano, parsley, rosemary, sage, sea salt, thyme, tumeric
Nuts & Seeds	Almonds, sunflower seeds, sesame seeds, walnuts, cashews, macadamia nuts, brazil nuts, pistachios
Beans & Legumes	Black beans, pinto beans, lentils, peas, kidney beans, azuki beans, butter beans
Grains	Rice, buckwheat, millet, sorghum, quinoa

Figure 4- *Hypoglycemia or low blood sugar symptoms*

Irritability relieved by eating	Forgetfulness
Lightheaded/Dizziness relieved by eating	Headaches (especially behind the right eye)
Fatigue (mental and/or physical) relieved by eating	Salt cravings

Figure 5- *Hyperglycemia or high blood sugar symptoms*

Fatigue after a meal	Getting sleepy after a meal
Not being able to concentrate after a meal	Frequent urination
Frequent hunger	Frequent/Increased thirst

Figure 6- *What not to eat*

Any food that you are allergic to.	Any food that you are sensitive to.
Wheat & Gluten	Non-organic Corn
Pasteurized and/or conventional dairy	Non-organic Soy
Genetically Modified Foods- Non-organic corn, soy, sugar beets, alfalfa, canola, etc.	Peanuts
	Unfermented Cauliflower
Fastfood	Soda, carbonated drinks, alcohol
Hydrogenated oils, partially hydrogentated oils, trans fats	

Figure 7- *Common and Major Stressors*

Frequent and/or extreme fluctuations in our Blood Sugar	Allowing our body to get too hot or too cold (extreme weather conditions)
Over-training	Emotional stress
Food Sensitivities	Pharmaceutical drugs
Synthetic vitamins and supplements	Not eating food with proper nutrient levels
Autoimmunity	Infection
Environmental chemicals, like BPA, pesticides, herbicides, smog, heavy metals	Conventional Dental work, especially mercury amalgam fillings and root canals
Recreational drugs, such as alcohol, tobacco	Dysbiosis & sub-clinical infections

Figure 8- *Common Signs of Stress*

Weight gain in the abdomen	High blood pressure
Depression	Anxiety
Insomnia	Waking up tired
Fatigue	Feeling worn down
Osteoporosis	Dysmenorrhea
Infertility	Loss of sex drive
Getting sick frequently	Low immune system
Memory lapses	Low learning abilities
Pain that won't go away	Mood Swings

How to measure your heart rate:

To measure your heart rate, locate your radial pulse or carotid pulse. The radial pulse can be found by pressing lightly on the thumb side of your wrist, just beneath the palm, on inside of the bone that connects the wrist to the root of the thumb. The carotid pulse can be found by touching the bone behind either ear and then sliding your fingers along the jaw line toward the side of your throat and applying light pressure into your neck. Once you've found your pulse, count the number of pulsations or beats over one minute. This is your resting heart rate in beats per minute. Optionally, you can count the number of pulsations or beats over 15 seconds and multiply it by 4 to estimate your heart rate in beats per minute (bpm).

Important concepts to remember:

- *If you have not exercised for an extended period of time or if you have never exercised, prepare the inside of your body first, then move on toward exercising the physical body.*

- *In the absence of trauma, your pain is usually caused by or promoted by internal dysfunction.*

- *Remember just because a food is labeled gluten-free, organic, or vegan does not mean that it is a quality food. There is a lot of junk food that carries those labels.*

- *Meat, fish, vegetables, and fruit will do more good than harm, and should be at the core of your diet.*

- *The truth is, that we all have an idea of what it takes to be healthy, we just need to listen to that part of us without the static of today's world drowning out the message.*

<u>YOUR HEALTH</u> IS IN <u>YOUR HANDS!</u>

RECOMMENDED READING TO TAKE YOUR HEALTH TO THE NEXT LEVEL:

Health:

Walking the Path to Health: How to continue in the right direction by Dr. Richard Robles

A follow up to The Path To Health, this book will focus on how to stay on the path to health. Once you have found the boundaries of your path, you will need to focus on identifying the moments when you may be straying from your path. It also contains practical solutions for some common problems people have with staying on the Path to Health.

Why Do I Still Have Thyroid Symptoms? When My Lab Tests Are Normal by Dr. Datis Kharrazian

> Dr. Kharrazian elaborates on the complexities of the way the body works on the inside. You will have a better understanding of how your body works and communicates on a deeper level. If you suffer from thyroid symptoms this book will give you a better understanding about why the problem usually isn't just with your thyroid. Also, check out his new book: *Why Isn't My Brain Working?*

Cleaning up your household environment:

The Honest Life by Jessica Alba

> This book will help you identify products and chemicals in your household environment. She does an excellent job of presenting the information in an easy to understand and practical way. When you are serious about removing the stress from your household environment, this book is a must read.

ADD, ADHD, Autism Spectrum Disorders, Dyslexia, and learning disabilities:

Disconnected Kids by Dr. Robert Melillo

Dr. Mellilo gives a detailed breakdown of proper brain development and what to look for functionally when things go wrong. This book will give you the tools to improve the brain health of yourself and your children. Functional balance of the brain is one of the best ways you can destress your nervous system. This book is a must read for all parents whether or not your child has a neurodegenerative condition.

Please visit us online for further recommended reading and other health information at:

www.myhealthmanual.com

Made in the USA
Lexington, KY
23 November 2016